What YOU Need To Know About Massage Therapy

A Helpful Book For Every Human Being

Levi G. Eckert

MYTHIC PEN PRESS
GREENVILLE, SC

TABLE OF CONTENTS

INTRODUCTION

In 2006, I had a life changing work accident: a thirty-foot fall from a high storage rack in a warehouse stock-room all the way down to the cement floor.

The impact with the concrete ground damaged my entire left side. Left hip, left wrist, and left head. A small sinus bone broke in the left side of my head, as well as my left wrist. The wrist break needed surgery, requiring a metal plate to heal the bone correctly. My spine, face, and right foot received nerve damage. Living was filled with pain and dysfunction for several years after the disabling injury.

I had to go to doctor and lawyer visits due to the injury happening at work. Physical therapy was critical in my wrist's recovery. My lawyer requested for me to get an MRI, but my doctor refused to do one. Without receiving a measurement of the damage to my spine, it wasn't taken care of properly. To this day, I have unmeasured nerve damage in my spine.

Damage sustained in the fall affected my memory, speech, and mobility. From that moment on I couldn't speak without stuttering and my memory felt like it was in a fog I couldn't see through. Scar tissue in my left wrist fused to some of the mechanical parts of my first two fingers and thumb.

My left hand had some dysfunction, my back caused electrical shock pains periodically, and headaches ruled my life. It took me a few weeks to be able to walk correctly and a few years to feel almost normal again.

Then it happened, after years of intense pain mixed with mental, emotional, and physical chal-lenges, a friend introduced me to chiropractic care and massage therapy. I was shy, nervous, hesitant, and uncomfortable about being touched by others, but I needed something to change.

Thanks to the chiropractor and massage therapist duo, my suffering decreased over time. It worked amazingly well together. The physical care truly blew my mind. Years of pain and disability began to lessen. Pain had been a part of my every day and almost every motion.

My health journey taught me a lot and it made me want to do something that I swore I would never do: go to school.

I've been an introvert my entire life. Being in school, being in public, public speaking, none of it came easy, but I had a feeling inside of me. I just knew I could help others the way I had been helped, so I built up my courage and pushed forward.

Next, I signed up for the massage therapy course at Greenville Tech. There I became one of the managers of the massage clinic and I made the Dean's list through the entire course. A small accomplishment, but it felt good to know I was heading in the right direction.

In 2012, I began working for a chiropractor's office. I started out as an introverted massage newbie with very little confidence. After ten years of serving the community that I live in, I've grown into a knowledgeable professional that cares about each person's massage results as if they were my own.

One of the big goals for this book is to educate people so everyone can receive the proper care at the right time with the best methods of massage available. This is all to help the body heal correctly, stay functional, and to keep a human's quality of life as high as possible for as long as possible.

I wrote this book to help *anyone* understand why

massage is helpful. No matter what level of familiarity a person has with massage, I strive to make it easy to see the importance of adding massage therapy to your self-care routine.

At some point during my health journey a notion came to mind. To eliminate pain in your life, you must understand it better. That's where this book comes in. It teaches what type of massage you need, why massage is helpful, and when you should get massage therapy. It also covers what can be massaged and what can't.

This book will give everyone a chance to under-stand why your body needs care and to take action against their physical problems before they cause long term damage.

Massage therapy is a great place to start for posi-tive physical change and the best way to under-stand what your body is going through.

ONE
MASSAGE THERAPY:
AN OVERVIEW

The first thing people usually wonder is, "Do I need massage therapy?"

Yes, you do. Your body needs massage therapy. Every physical, mental, and emotional situation that you endure can cause your muscles to respond with tension.

If you feel pain or stress and let it go untreated, your muscles and joints could begin to lose their physical ability to function at their best.

The longer your muscles stay tight or affected by pain and dysfunction, the less likely they will operate at 100%. Massage therapy helps keep your muscles and joints flexible, strong, and able by attending to the soft tissues of the human body.

Massage therapy uses therapeutic touch and different pressures on the body to relax, relieve pain, improve joint mobility, and to improve health.

1.1: MASSAGE BENEFITS

Massage can provide the following benefits:

- Decreased stress
- Relaxed muscles
- Ease of pain and aches
- Can relieve headaches
- Decreased tension
- Increased blood flow
- Increased nutrient absorption
- Increased immune system response
- Increased endorphins (the "feel good" hormone)
- Improved joint mobility and flexibility
- Filter organs remove waste more efficiently
- Moisturized skin
- Improved body awareness and pain acknowledge-ment
- Body education from a trained massage therapist
- Can improve sleep

Massage therapy can do a lot of good. One of the most influential benefits of massage is increased blood flow. Nearly every component of the human body can improve with greater access to blood.

On a normal day, white blood cells move slowly on their own. With massage therapy, the immune system can be encouraged to move quicker.

As your blood flow increases, your kidneys and liver are able to filter out waste from the blood quicker and more efficiently.

During your massage session, the therapist may touch muscles or skin that is more tender than you expected. Your body awareness and pain acknowledgement grows as you are touched with massage, and it teaches you to care for the less critical issues as they appear.

If you absolutely **knew** what would bring a positive physical change to your life, whether it was massage, physical activity, or another type of care, would you push your health journey to embrace it?

When we know what we need, it's much easier to take that step to make change.

<u>Fun note</u>: When your body performs a good wellness routine, the muscular tension melts away easier.

1.2: What can be massaged?

Before your first massage, it is most helpful to know what *can* be massaged. Every working part of the human body can benefit from physical attention.

Everything can be massaged unless there is a health condition that prevents the therapy from being applied safely.

Here is a general list of body parts that can be assisted through massage therapy.

The Human Head

Scalp

The scalp has muscles around it that can be relaxed with therapeutic massage. Head muscles can hold tension just like any other muscle can. Some tight scalp muscles may cause headaches.

Sinus cavities run throughout the head and can be assisted with massage.

Neck

Your neck muscles support your head. We often use our necks in ways they are not designed for, like looking down at a cell phone for hours, driving too long, or sitting at the computer for too long.

Massage therapy can help the neck to relax, flex, and support, allowing it to do its job with less restriction.

Face

Massage therapy can help face muscles to relax and assist the sinuses. It may surprise you how much we use our face muscles involuntarily. When we experience deep emotions or squint from the bright sun, our facial muscles are being used. Our face's need care to relax from all we put them through.

Overused face muscles can become very tight, causing headaches, jaw pain, or even disorders with the jaw.

Jaw

The jaw muscles can be used too much and could require more care than you would expect. Talking too much, chewing, or clenching your teeth can lead to tension that massage therapy can aid.

Some therapists have extra training to work with the internal mouth muscles to help with jaw related issues.

Example: TMJD (Temporo-Mandibular Joint Disorder), commonly referred to as TMJ, is a jaw condition. The jaw can be affected by grinding or clenching teeth, chewing too much on one side of the mouth, or arthritis. A lot of overuse types of motions.

TMJ disorders may include:

- Pain in the jaw on one or both sides
- Discomfort during chewing
- Aching around the ear
- Facial pain
- Jaw operation difficulty
- Arthritis

The head, face, neck, and jaw can improve with the benefits of massage therapy greatly. Relaxing the muscles of the head and face could help you to breath, sleep, and relax deeper. Even the ears can relax.

UPPER BODY

Chest

Massage to the chest muscles can help the shoulders, neck, and upper back to relax. These groups of muscles are all connected and work together. If the chest muscles become too tight, it can then roll the shoulders forward affecting the neck and upper back negatively.

In some cases, the chest can be sore after having an episode with a lung illness or excessive coughing. Therapeutic massage could be helpful for recovery by assisting the muscles associated with coughing.

Shoulders

These hard-working muscles can get pulled to the

front of the body by the chest muscles. Tight chest and neck muscles can restrict the full range of motion (ROM) of the shoulders.

Many muscle groups around the shoulders can cause problems over the long term if tension or pain is ignored.

Massage therapy can improve shoulder ROM and ability. Shoulders work hard and sometimes need to be tenderized by a professional for them to continue their tasks with less complaints. Arm stretches may be applied by the therapist.

Elbow

This may seem like a strange place to target for relief, but massage therapy can help by improving mobility of skin and connective tissue. Several muscles connect to the elbow that can benefit from release of tension.

Most joints have the ability to have tendonitis, but it's most common in the elbows, shoulders, and knees. Tendonitis means tendon inflammation. People that use their hands with a lot of strength tend to get this issue. This is classified as a repetitive use problem.

Tennis Elbow and Golfer's Elbow are common overuse and strain issues, which ice and rest help a lot with. Massage can assist the elbow's function once the inflammation has reduced.

Arms and Hands

Usually one of the most used body parts, these can

definitely benefit from massage. The more a human's body is used, the more care it needs to stay healthy, happy, and able. Arms and hands are no exception.

Massage can help the hand muscles to relax and function better. The therapist may also know a couple stretches to apply. Hands that have received damage need to be addressed with therapeutic massage. It can help to loosen up scar tissues, relax the hard-working muscles, and could mobilize stuck connective tissue.

Hands can be damaged easily and often. As we go through life, our hands can get hurt in a variety of ways. Car door slams, knife cuts, scrapes, stabs, gouges, broken bones, jammed fingers. (Come to think of it, I've had all of these.)

Don't ignore your most used body parts. Even with no pain present, working muscles still deserve positive attention and care.

CORE: ABDOMEN & BACK

Abdomen (the belly)

The core abdomen area is composed of several layers of flat muscles that pull in different directions. Core muscles need to be strong to support the low back. A weak core means the lower back will struggle over time.

Haven't gone to the bathroom in a while? Massage may be able to help move things along, if you are comfortable having your abdomen massaged lightly.

Mayan Abdominal Massage is a good example of a long-standing tradition of massage to the belly or womb. Belly massage can improve digestion, can boost the immune system, decrease PMS symptoms, and can also release emotional and physical stress or trauma.

Back

Many muscles run up and down the spine, across the back, and around the sides. These muscles support posture mostly. *Any* muscle that supports posture can benefit from relaxation.

Massage can target the muscles along the spine, shoulder blades, low, middle, and upper back. There are 24 vertebrae in the spine. The spinal muscles that support those bones can be addressed with regularly scheduled massage therapy.

LOWER BODY

Glutes

Aka the butt, or Gluteus Maximus, Medius, and Minimus.

These muscles allow us to sit, stand, walk, run, jump, and squat. Massage therapy can relax the strong layers of these muscles.

The glutes are highly used for motion and stability.

<u>Fun note</u>: Gluteus maximus is the largest muscle in the body.

These strong muscles cover over the sciatic nerve that runs down the leg. Massage therapy can reduce the effects of some sciatica cases.

Sciatica is a condition that occurs when the sciatic nerve is pinched. This usually causes numbness, tingling, weakness, or pain.

Massage therapy can work with sciatica, but depending on the cause the results may vary. If the issue is brought on by spinal misalignment, herniated disc, or bone spur then massage may have limited results.

Knee

Our knees can be affected by the struggles of our hips and feet. Massage therapy can reduce connective tissue restriction around the knee and improve flexibility.

When you feel an issue with any joint, get it worked with as soon as you can. Joints work hard enough without pain coming in and trying to take over.

Massage therapists may perform some stretches with the leg to assess and assist the knee's motion.

Legs

Long appendages that come from the hips. Massage therapy is excellent for the legs. The strong leg muscles need physical attention, especially if you have a job or hobby that uses them a lot.

Your massage therapist may perform leg stretches. Just remember to relax and be vocal if you need the therapist to stop any stretch for any reason.

Hamstrings, calves, quads, shin, and groin area. Massage therapy can be performed along the entire leg. The groin remains covered when that work is necessary.

Ankles

Our ankles can suffer from a range of problems due to running, jumping, landing, standing, or twisting. Massage therapy can improve motion of ankles by reducing resistant connective tissue around the joint.

Feet

Massage can help remove inflammation in the feet as well as loosen tense muscles and stuck connective tissue.

Important: Keep good feet hygiene in mind when seeking a foot massage. Clean feet are a necessity. A massage therapist can turn away a client if their hygiene is not properly taken care of.

Plantar fasciitis, inflammation in the foots' connective tissue (fascia), can be caused by old or poorly supportive shoes and too much time spent on your feet for a long term.

Tip #1: Treat the feet well.

Your feet get you every place you need to go. Think of how much you put your feet through as you give them some care. Give them an Epsom salt soak, get them massaged, and keep your feet happy and able.

Other Areas

I named some general parts of the body that can be massaged, but pretty much any muscle can be assisted with therapeutic touch.

1.3: HEALTH CONDITIONS

If you are seeking a massage for a certain health condition, you may need to do some online research first. You should call and ask your chosen therapist if they can accommodate you and your needs before scheduling a session.

Massage therapy can be good for some conditions and should be avoided with others. Here are some common conditions that massage therapists come in contact with.

Acne

A very common skin condition. The therapist may wear medical gloves with this and many other skin conditions. Excessive, inflamed, or "angry" acne is avoided. Touching irritated skin can cause more irritation and is best left alone. Massage can still be beneficial while avoiding the skin issue.

Carpal Tunnel Syndrome

Can be caused by heavy computer use, device use, or other repetitive motions. This condition usually comes from a pinching or pressure on the median arm nerve or nerve pressures from the neck.

Massage therapy can assist the muscles that are involved with those nerves and release muscular tension from them.

In some cases, the condition may need surgery to improve. Massage therapy can be helpful after the surgery heals.

Ask your doctor if it's safe for you to get massage therapy.

Fibromyalgia

Muscle fiber pain. There is no known cause. This is a long-lasting disorder that causes pain, tenderness, fatigue, and trouble sleeping.

Massage therapy is a great option to improve sleep, reduce pain, and elevate mood.

Headaches

Headaches can be caused by tight muscles in the neck, face, shoulders, chest, and back. High stress, leaning your head forward for too long, or sinus problems can also lead to headaches.

Other causes of headaches include chemical or hormone imbalance, dehydration, poor spinal alignment, blood pressure issues, or detoxing.

Massage therapy can relax the muscles that cause headaches and can improve neck flexibility.

Osteoporosis

This condition causes weakened bone structure in the elderly. Most commonly seen in females. The bones become porous and easier to break with less effort. Massage therapy can usually be performed lightly, depending on the severity of the disease.

Important: If you have concerns about the massage pressure, you can ask your massage therapist to use light pressure.

With massage, the blood flow increases, mood improves, and waste can be removed through the filter organs easier. Very positive things for elderly patients.

Sciatica

Sciatica is most commonly caused by tight hip (butt) muscles, spinal misalignment, or herniated discs. Most common with sit down jobs and driving.

Sitting too long can create discomfort or pain that can be felt going down one or both legs. Some people also experience numbness or tingling in the legs or feet.

Sciatica can linger if not cared for.

Massage therapy can reduce hip muscle tension and improve flexibility, but further care from another specialist may be needed. Check with your doctor.

Tendonitis

Occurs when a tendon that connects a muscle to a bone becomes inflamed. Overused joints can suffer from this. Apply ice to the affected area and give it plenty of rest.

A supportive brace can be used to restrict excessive

motion and swelling of the affected joint.

Massage can help the affected area by improving circulation, relaxing muscle, and assisting the removal of inflammation. It also helps to improve motion to the joint.

1.4: MEDICATIONS

Medications are used for very specific purposes. Most medications have side effects and each person can react to them differently. It's important for you to know what the side effects of your medications are.

It's easy to forget the small details with long term medications. Some common medications create muscular tension as a side effect. If you *know* that your medicine causes muscular tension, then it could be help-ful to counter that with massage before it causes dis-comfort, pain, or dysfunction.

A medication's response to the human system can vary by person. Some people can be extremely sensitive or resistant to chemical medications.

Check with your doctor to determine if massage is safe for your condition and medications.

Important: If you have a heart issue and are **not** on medication for it, massage should be **avoided**. Massage increases blood flow and could cause an untreated condition to act up. Please, keep your medical conditions under control to receive the full benefits of massage.

Pain Medication

When people feel pain, they take pain medication. It's common. Pain medicine helps to relieve the feeling of pain, but when you don't feel the pain anymore; it's much easier to damage the affected area without realizing it.

Overusing a painful area, even if the pain is hidden by medication, could lead to inflammation or injury, causing it to take *more* time to heal the issue.

It's easy to feel like medicine can fix anything when it relieves pain, but we all know that chemicals can't massage sore muscles, stretch, improve flexibility, or work out knots.

Try to be thoughtful of your medications and their side effects.

What this means: when you are taking pain medication, give the affected area time to rest. It's hard for the body to heal when it struggles and experiences pain consistently.

Give your body the opportunity to heal.

Tip #2: Making your injured body parts struggle may not be helpful.

1.5: TRAUMA AND MASSAGE

Traumatic events can push our lives in unexpected directions. Massage therapy can help trauma victims to relax on a deeper level over time.

Types of trauma:

- Physical
- Mental
- Emotional
- Sexual
- Dental
- Surgical

Traumas are not easy battles to win. Progress can be made towards healing with help from a trusted massage therapist and other healthcare specialists. Trauma victims need more time and patience to fight their battles.

If you have been through a trauma, ask a doctor if massage therapy would help. Traumas of all types can cause high-level tension without the victim realizing that it's even happening.

No matter what type of trauma a person receives, the body responds with tension or guarding, exactly what massage therapy can assist with.

There is always a mental portion involved when

overcoming trauma. A trained and licensed psychologist may be helpful for even deeper results.

Working towards a positive mindset is difficult in the face of pain and struggle, but it's worth fighting for.

Remember: Recovery takes patience, persistence, and understanding. Be kind to yourself.

Sometimes hearing that massage therapy could be helpful is an unwelcome piece of news for a person. Even if someone is completely set against seeing a trained professional for any reason, it's still good to lessen their traumas on whatever level they *are* comfortable with.

I've been through traumatic events myself and I want other victims to know that there are helpful solutions out there. You just have to be willing to seek them.

It's not where you want to be, but you can still make progress.

Ask your doctor about any health concerns.

You're probably saying, "He said to see my doctor a LOT." It's true. I did. Doctors are trained in diagnosis and have the tools to point you in the right direction. Sometimes NO massage therapy is the answer. Both you and the massage therapist need to know that.

1.6: WHEN <u>NOT</u> TO SEE A MASSAGE THERAPIST

Massage therapy should avoid sensitive health issues because the physical treatment could make the issue worse to some degree. In some cases, NO massage is the best choice.

Some problems cannot be helped by massage therapy or should not be treated with touch, such as:

- Unmedicated blood pressure problems
- Infections of skin or blood
- Open wounds
- Deep bruises
- Major swelling or inflammation
- Pitting edema
- Broken bones
- Lice
- High fever
- Right after major surgery
- Internal pain
- Advanced organ failure
- Contagious disease

Talk to your doctor about any health conditions to determine if massage is safe for you. Factual information from an educated professional can deepen your understanding of the condition.

Tip #3: The more you know, the less you guess.

1.7: MINORS AND MASSAGE THERAPY

Many massage businesses or therapists limit their patients to 18 or older, but the truth is a human of any age can be massaged. Finding a therapist that accommodates minors will make your rambunctious youth's life much easier and their future brighter.

It's important for kids to learn how to avoid future problems by getting their aches and pains assessed and worked with professionally. Any child that plays on a sports team of any kind can improve with the benefits from massage.

The parent or guardian may sit in the massage room during the session. For young children, a massage session should be between ten and twenty minutes. A full hour would be too much for a young person.

Teenagers are bigger and should be able to handle more time. Thirty minutes to an hour should be appropriate for their session.

A lot of kids are ticklish, which is a challenge for the therapist to overcome. Just know that the therapist isn't trying to tickle on purpose.

Asking questions to the therapist may help you feel more comfortable about them working on your child.

If our injuries are given excellent care as early as possible, it could limit how much the issue affects us in the future. When kids learn how to care for their hurt parts, we all suffer less. Parents included.

1.8: ELDERLY AND MASSAGE THERAPY

It's good for every human to get massage therapy no matter their age unless a condition or disease prevents treatment.

Massage therapists require a health history before working on any person. Make certain to be honest and clear about any medications and health issues that the elderly client has. Share as much information as you can with your therapist.

Important note: Some medications may affect the way a person feels pressure or temperature.

Example of an elderly condition to be careful with: **Osteoporosis** can weaken the bones. Most commonly found in females but males can still be affected. Caution is required with massage pressure. Massage can be helpful with this condition if the therapist knows and understands their client's needs and restrictions.

Massage can assist the elderly in positive ways, like:

- Improved circulation
- lymph drainage
- assists nutrient absorption
- improved skin health
- improved joint mobility
- human touch: sometimes just being touched by another caring human can be helpful.

Improved circulation is one of the more helpful aspects. It assists with removal of inflammation, lymph, and other built-up materials in the body. Every human body needs their waste material removed from the body. It's a necessary process that is improved with massage therapy.

A relaxing massage is most common for an elderly client. Light to medium pressure is usually recommended.

It can be good for the elderly to receive some light stretching if there are no serious restrictions. If there are any joint mobility concerns, make sure to tell the massage therapist before or during the session. The therapist can be more careful when stretching those concerning areas.

Many elderly people that live a more sedentary life could be extra tender and stiff. A few sessions may be necessary to relieve some of the long-term aches and pains. Remember, a massage can assist the human body's ability to rest, restore, and recover.

Ask your regular physician if massage is ok for you. They know your medications and health issues and can determine if massage will be helpful or harmful. Massage therapists cannot diagnose illness or injury, or prescribe medications.

1.9: PHYSICAL LIMITATIONS

People that live life in handicapped ways need as much massage therapy as anyone else, maybe more so. Any physical limitation will put a strain on the surrounding muscles and functions.

Massage therapy can assist people who use a wheelchair, or crutches, wear a protective boot, or bone-break cast, or are bed bound.

Any muscles that can't be used or properly supportive needs to be massaged and assisted with a much-needed circulation boost.

Some massage therapists may go their entire careers without working on a physically handicapped person. When you seek massage therapy for a handicapped person, make sure to call and confirm that the therapist is knowledgeable of the specific handicap, understands how to assist you, and can accommodate any limitations associated.

TWO
Finding A Massage Therapist

This section should help you to learn more about what you are seeking from a therapeutic massage, that way you will know what to look for when you search for your therapist.

How do I know what kind of massage therapy I am looking for?

That's a good question. You have to start somewhere and it's usually a safe bet to find a relaxing massage therapist to enter the world of massage first. You will gain some understanding of how massage feels and what to expect. You may even fall asleep on the table.

If an injury or pain has you looking for a massage therapist, it could be more beneficial to start with a deep tissue therapist. It's important to note that deep tissue therapy can leave the affected area more sore after a session. This is due to its focused techniques. Even with the soreness it does help to make deeper, longer-lasting changes.

Results vary for each session. The fact remains the same for everyone, the body needs consistent maintenance, and massage therapy is the best place to assist with positive physical change.

What type of massage do I need?

Know what you are seeking from a massage. Knowing what your body needs can waste less money and time on treatments that may not help much. Many massage styles feel good, but they may not be what you need to make a bigger change.

No one likes putting money in a vending machine just to have it keep your money and what you hoped you would get in return: Peanut butter cheese crackers. Yum. Oh, I mean feeling better for longer.

There are different types of massage therapies and therapists. Find out what a therapist specializes in before you schedule a session.

<u>Example</u>: If you want deep pressure. Knowing that a relaxing massage is usually light to medium pressure could help point you in the right direction. If a therapist specializes in relaxing massage, their pressure may not go as deep as you want or need. Make sure your therapist has that ability you seek before you schedule an appointment with them.

Disappointment brews when expectations are not

met or fully understood. Take the time to find out what you need and match it with a therapist with the appropriate skills.

Some massage therapists offer a consultation before scheduling a massage, which allows you and the therapist to determine if their skills match your goals.

Use the right tool for the job. Find a therapist with the skills to get the physical change you are seeking.

Tip #4: Use the right tool for the job.

If you have any concerns about massage therapy, speak to your doctor. Physicians are trained to determine if massage is safe for many conditions.

2.1: MASSAGE STYLES

Swedish massage and deep tissue massage are two of the most commonly practiced styles that a therapist can specialize in. It's good to know these for when you're searching for the best massage therapist for you.

I rely on these the most to help clients recover from stress and pain.

RELAXATION (AKA SWEDISH) MASSAGE

The most commonly referred to type of massage is Relaxation, or Swedish, Massage. When someone thinks of the word massage, this is usually what they imagine. This modality relaxes the body, making a client more likely to fall asleep during this session. Relaxing massage techniques are the most helpful for stress reduction.

This type of massage promotes good circulation. With good circulation, your organs can filter the waste materials out better and oxygen, hydration, and nutrients can affect more muscle as the improved circulation moves.

Important: Relaxing massage is not usually done with deep or heavy pressure. It is usually a light to medium pressure style. With that said, there are many heavy-handed therapists out there. If heavy pressure is what you seek, make sure the therapist can meet that expectation before scheduling a session.

Swedish massage sessions can be full-body oriented. During the session, the patient will lay on their back, front, or both, splitting the time between them. Some therapists may lay a client on their side to perform a specific technique.

Relaxing sessions are most commonly thirty, sixty, or ninety minutes.

DEEP TISSUE THERAPY

Deep Tissue Therapy is a goal-focused massage for painful or tight muscular areas. This method focuses on the deeper layers of muscles and connective tissues, which helps to decrease pain and tension as well as increase mobility and function.

A deep tissue massage session could spend most or all of the time focused on the chosen area. It's easy to spend thirty minutes on one region of the body.

Trigger point work and stretching could be involved. Communication between patient and therapist is *necessary* to obtain the best results.

"That's the spot. I feel that going up to my head. How do you know where those pressure spots are?" said an amazed client.

"Ow, that's tender," the same client said a moment later.

Deep tissue massage can be a little painful or sore, but it's necessary to ease pressure in muscle groups, nerves, and joints. It can even help to soften tough scar tissue.

Trigger Points (TP) are small, knotted portions of a muscle. The affected muscle can be *very* tight and feel like a small ball, rock, or knot under the skin. TPs can affect the nerves around them.

<u>Example</u>: There is a common TP in the upper trapezius muscle that connects the shoulder to the neck. Pressure applied here could cause numbness, tingling, or pain to travel down the arm or up into the head.

When a therapist puts pressure on a TP, pain can be felt in and around it in most cases. It can also feel like the pain is moving away from where the pressure is applied.

TPs do not normally go away on their own and can be more tender as they receive massage.

Trigger Points can go through periods of being active, which produces pain on its own, and dormant, which only hurts when pressed or triggered.

The two states of a Trigger Point:

- Active: You may feel pain in and around the trigger point or it may shoot pain without any prompting. Pressure in an active TP may amplify the sensation.
- Dormant: The TP exists but is only noticed when pressure is applied.

One of Deep Tissue Therapy's main goals is to find and defeat these evil doers, er, I mean, tense muscle and nerve bundles. Most muscles have the ability to be affected by TPs, even jaw muscles.

DEEP TISSUE METHODS

Myofascial Release

A kind of deep tissue therapy that focuses on releasing the stuck connective tissue around muscles and joints.

<u>Example</u>: The skin around the lower back can get stuck to the muscles and the spinal bones if you have to sit for a long period of time without relief of position for a long term.

These stuck tissues can become dehydrated over time and eventually restrict motion and blood to the area. Deep tissue therapists can help mobilize this connective material to keep all the hydration and blood flowing through as it should.

Neuromuscular Therapy

A kind of deep tissue therapy that focuses on relieving muscle pressure from nerves. Trigger Point work falls under this category.

Personally, I do a ton of Trigger Point work. It's tender work that pays off by providing greater relief and better function.

2.2: HOW TO MAXIMIZE YOUR DEEP TISSUE RESULTS

Deep Tissue Therapy is a goal-oriented type of massage and is most helpful over several consecutive sessions.

One to two 30-minute sessions per week for two to eight weeks. Or...

One one-hour session per week for two to eight weeks.

These are the usual ranges of care that I use for specific issue treatment. Even when you feel great, a one-hour massage every month can keep pain from returning by staying aware of any physical issues.

For a thirty-minute deep tissue session, I like to focus on one to two points of concern.

For an hour-long session, I allow time for two to four issues to be addressed. Every session varies.

It takes time and effort for the massage techniques to work the tension away and to make a deep change.

Tip #5: Consistency is the key to noticeable change.

<u>Example</u>: You go to the gym once and you exercise one time.

How much change do you think you made with one effort?

How about 100 efforts?

The key to a properly working body and a pain-free future is consistency of self-care, like: Massage therapy, being physical, rest, stretching, hydration, deep breathing, positivity, and time to reflect and grow from what we've learned.

2.3: OTHER MASSAGE STYLES

These are some other massage styles that you may or may not have heard of. Therapists that specialize in these styles are easiest found online or by word of mouth. Trying a new type of therapy may be helpful to get the results that you're seeking.

Lymphatic

A gentle touch massage to stimulate the flow of lymph (white blood cells) and assist removal of excess fluids. Often used with injury, surgery, or cancer.

Sports

A blend of relaxing massage, deep tissue, and stretching. It is most helpful for athletic people that use their bodies to their highest ability regularly.

Integrated

A combination of two or more massage styles. Relaxing and Deep Tissue combination is my favorite and what I use most.

Thai

Similar to assisted yoga with added massage techniques. You may lie on a mat rather than a massage table. Clients wear loose, flexible clothing as in yoga.

Cupping

Use of suction cups. Helps to bring blood to the surface or into tight muscles. Can leave bruise-colored circles, which are usually pain free. Tell your therapist if any device they use hurts.

Chair (or seated)

Massage performed on a massage chair or in a seated position. Mostly focused on the upper back, neck, and arms.

Hot stone

A relaxing massage using smooth stones that have been heated by water. The stones can be placed on the body or used with massage strokes. Hot stones are just as they sound: very hot.

Important: Talk to your therapist if the stones are too hot. You don't want to be burned. You may trust your therapist to know when to move them, but massage therapists cannot feel what you feel. So, please, speak up if you feel something negative.

Reflexology

Massage and pressure point work with the feet or hands, sometimes the ears. The entire session could be foot- or hand-focused. These therapists are called reflexologists.

Prenatal

Massage for pregnant women, usually performed with the client on her side. This massage is done to avoid any unwanted pressure on the abdomen. The therapist may use a pillow for the pregnant woman's head, leg, and arm to rest on.

Important: Some people believe that it is best to wait until the 2nd trimester before getting massage therapy. The first trimester can be a sensitive time for some pregnancies.

Shiatsu

A type of massage therapy originating from Japan that involves pressing specific points in the body to reduce tension by improving circulation.

Craniosacral Therapy

A gentle touch therapy in which the practitioner applies hands-on techniques to the soft tissues, fascia, bones, and cerebrospinal fluid that passes through the central nervous system.

Important: CST has been used to treat a variety of physical and psychological conditions. Talk with your therapist to learn if they can work with your condition before scheduling a session.

These are the most common massage styles. There are more types out there, but we'll focus mostly on relaxation and deep tissue.

Massage therapy, in general, can assist in preventing injuries and connective tissue issues. If you have already been injured, massage can assist your healing journey.

2.4: CHOOSE THE RIGHT METHOD FOR YOU

Put some time into finding a good massage therapist. The correct care for your goal could change your life, but it's possible to get the wrong massage at the wrong time.

Be aware of the cautions.

WRONG TYPES OF CARE

Some folks have told me they had a bad experience for their first massage due to expectations not being met. The better you understand what your body needs, the easier it is to find a massage therapist that can meet your expectations. Most people don't realize that there are different types of massage therapy and can get the wrong type of physical care for their issue.

<u>Example 1</u>: Getting a relaxing massage when you're recovering from a recent car accident. It can feel nice, but it won't assist with making significant changes that are needed to recover from such a physical trauma.

Deep Tissue Therapy can help improve the mobility and function of recovering areas far more than a relaxing massage.

<u>Example 2</u>: Receiving a deep tissue massage too soon after an injury could cause excessive inflammation and

extra damage to the affected region. Only light massage is recommended on an inflamed area. If the area has too much inflammation, massage should be *avoided* until the inflammation has lessened.

Depending on the injury, you may need to wait two to six days before the affected area can be massaged.

When you find a good therapist that understands you and your physical issues, it's easier for you to relax and trust their assessments and techniques. Bear in mind that it can take several sessions to make a bigger difference.

When massage therapy is added to a regular exercise and stretching routine, a person can stay strong and able for longer, with the possibility of receiving fewer injuries along the way.

Every human is unique and carries their stress and pain differently.

Patience and understanding guides us through the darkness of pain.

If you have been getting massage therapy and feel like you aren't making any progress toward your goal, it's perfectly fine to find another therapist. Think of it as trying a different tool to get a different result.

Example: Would you take your car's transmission problem to someone that only does auto body work? The work doesn't align with your goal. You may be satisfied with how your car may look now, but the transmission problem is still there.

Both mechanics work on cars, but their goals are

different.

Tip #6: The ability of each massage therapist varies.

Take your time to find the right therapy for you.

"That massage didn't help very much." Many people say when their massage session results don't match their goal.

It can happen. Try to make sure your therapist under-stands what type of massage you need. If you're not certain, ask more questions about what you feel before, during, and after a massage. It is crucial that your therapist understands your physical issues as deeply as possible.

Clear communication between patient and therapist is a *must*.

Remember: It's ok to ask your therapist to make adjustments to the session to further improve your comfort and results. If you're too cold, hot, or uncomfortable. These small frustrations can decrease your ability to relax well for a therapeutic massage and could diminish good results.

Also, if you want more or less pressure, more time spent with pressure in a trigger point, or if you want a body part avoided or focused on for a variety of reasons, communicate that to your therapist.

Example 1: "I have a cut on my arm. Watch out for it, please."

Example 2: "Can you work on my face, feet, or hands?"

Face, feet, and hands are special request areas that

should be discussed before the session. Each therapist's routine will differ.

2.5: How to Find a Massage Therapist

Finding your therapist can take a little trial and error. Keep trying until you find the one that works the best for you and your needs.

Online Searches

The best way to find the specific type of massage therapist that you need. Typing the words 'Massage Therapy' and the name of your city can bring up plenty of options.

Word of Mouth

Reviews from friends and family are also a great way to find a good therapist. The big reminder with this method is that what works for your friend or family may not work for you. If that is the case, don't give up. Just try the next therapist on your list.

Hospital Referrals

Sometimes when people get injured or have an accident, the hospital may give a referral to get massage, chiropractic, or another type of care. Not all chiropractic offices do massage, so it may help to ask for a massage referral as well.

Doctor Recommendation

Some doctors may recommend that you seek a massage therapist. They may give you options or send you out into the world to find one on your own.

2.6: SETTINGS FOR MASSAGE THERAPY

Massage therapy can be performed in almost any location. Public or private. These are common professional settings that you could receive a massage at.

Massage Office

A business where massage therapy is provided. Usually with a peaceful aspect to it.

Chiropractor's Office

This is a doctor's office. Make sure your chiropractor provides massage therapy. Chiropractic and massage work together to treat physical ailments by targeting the bones and muscles. Tense musculature does not allow for smooth adjustments.

Spa

Classic full spa treatment. Spas usually have a massage therapist and various other spa treatments available. Spas do facial treatments, body treatments, massage therapy, and more.

A Therapist's Home

Some therapists operate out of their home.

Public Event

Chair massages are great for public events and can be performed outdoors at festivals, fairs, events, businesses, the beach, etc. Patrons stay clothed during a chair massage.

2.7: BEFORE YOUR FIRST MASSAGE

These are some things that need to be done and spoken about before the massage happens.

Health History

These forms are necessary to be filled out for massage therapy to be performed. A therapist should know any medical conditions you have. Some health issues need to be avoided with massage and it's important for you and your therapist to both know that.

Be honest. List medications that you are on.

Some medications cause changes in a person's ability to feel pressure, temperature, or pain, which could cause discomfort after the massage. The client would only realize that later when their medication has worn off.

The more we all know, the better the results.

Allergies

List things you are allergic to. Some people have sensitivities to certain massage lotions, creams, or oils. A good massage therapist usually has an alternative lotion just in case.

If you want to bring your own lotion, ask your therapist if it's ok first. They may have an allergy to certain products themselves.

If you do decide to bring your own lotion to your

session, please make sure the bottle is in good condition.

Good Hygiene

Practice good hygiene before getting massage therapy. It's easy for a strong aroma to overpower a small massage room. Try to be mindful of strong odors. Too much perfume or cologne can be just as bad as a negative smell.

Please be mindful of all aromas.

The Bathroom Talk

So, now you know what you need. You've found your therapist and you're waiting in the lobby for your appointment time. It may not seem like a big deal, but try to use the bathroom before a massage.

Lying down and being massaged can cause you to have the need to go to the bathroom. If you have to go and you choose not to, it could make you very uncomfortable. I, myself, have experienced this. I didn't speak up about my discomfort and I suffered. It isn't an enjoyable situation and It's best to be avoided.

If you have to get up to use the bathroom during a massage session, it hurts the quality, the time, and continuity of the flow. Redressing, going to the bathroom, coming back, and trying to relax again takes time away from your session.

For a smoother, better experience use the bathroom before your massage.

Long Hair

If you have long hair, do your best to keep it out of the way. High ponytails or buns are the best in my opinion. A hair wrap is a good option as well.

Most people don't enjoy lotion in their hair.

Jewelry

It's a good idea to remove necklaces and other jewelry around the regions you want massaged. Jewelry can get in the way and take away from the massage experience.

And again, most people don't like lotion on their precious gems and such.

Friendly Phone Reminder

Don't forget to turn your phone volume down and any alarms off while you are getting a massage. They can be quite loud and disruptive in a small, quiet room.

Your massage loses helpfulness when you or the therapist have to repeatedly deal with a device for any reason. Try to relax. You deserve some time for yourself.

Before the Massage

The therapist may ask you what your goal is, what is in pain, or if there is anything you need to avoid or focus on. You should have a small conversation about any health concerns and your massage goal.

Tell the therapist what you want for your session.

Example: Full body, or focus on head, neck and shoulders only, or low back and legs only. Share what you can with your therapist so they understand your situation as well as possible. Then they can formulate a care plan in their head.

Getting a full body massage is not the same as getting a deep tissue session. Deep tissue is a focused, goal type of massage. Relaxation style is usually a full body massage with no specific focus.

With a full body massage, the therapist will tell you which way to lay on the massage table. Face up or face down. About halfway through the massage, the therapist will want you to turn over to work on the other side of your body.

The therapist will lift the sheet slightly to allow you to move around without dragging the sheet off, keeping you draped appropriately.

With a deep tissue session, you go over what muscles or pain issues you want the therapist to work on. Then the therapist will tell you which way to lie on the massage table to work on the specified areas. Face up, face down, side-lying, or seated.

Get on the Table

The therapist steps out of the room. Now it's time to get comfortable.

There may be a sheet to get under. Some offices use medical gowns, robes, or shorts.

Undress to your level of comfort. Most commonly; people undress down to their underwear or sportswear. Some people may prefer to be fully nude, which is fine. Draping is applied to cover the massage recipient to keep their privates private.

I prefer for my clients to wear flexible sports clothes. It allows for many different types of stretches and techniques to be performed while you stay well-covered.

The therapist will knock on the door. You can respond with a cool phrase, like: "I'm ready!" or "Come in."

If you are sitting on a massage chair, make sure you're comfortable. The massage chair is adjustable, and the therapist can adjust it to how you need it.

2.8: WHAT TO EXPECT IN A MASSAGE SESSION

This is to help give you an inside view as to what a massage session can be like. Every massage session will vary. There are a lot of factors that go into building a massage session.

During Massage

Every therapist starts their sessions differently. You could start face up or face down on the massage table, or maybe even on your side. Your therapist may ask you about the pressure they are applying. Be honest please. Massage can be sore work to start out, but as the skin and muscle tissues relax, the tenderness can lessen.

The therapist will perform many massage techniques to relax the skin, muscles, and connective tissues. They may do some stretches for your arms, legs, hips, or neck during your session. Be verbal with what you feel, the therapist can't feel the pain or discomfort you may be feeling. Everyone's ability to stretch differs. Let the words out: "more," "less," or "ouchie."

Try your best to relax when someone else is stretching you, it's a different experience than stretching your own stuff.

Allow the therapist to mobilize your appendages.

Some people try to help with certain stretches, and it may cause a muscle pull if the muscle is unhealthy. Try to relax. If the stretch is painful, tell the therapist and they could stop the stretch if needed.

Communication is a big theme in care and recovery.

Your therapist may ask about your self-care routine.

Self-care is anything that you do to improve your own physical, mental, or emotional health.

Stretching, exercise, warm soaks, relaxation, restorative vacations, and more are considered to be self-care.

The End of the Session

Now the session is over. Some therapists wipe the excess lotion or oil off of their client, some do not. You can ask to have them remove the lotion if you feel it's too much. They may use a towel or some type of alcohol wipe.

You may receive a small amount of water from your therapist as you exit the massage room. Drinking extra water is usually encouraged after a massage.

After the Massage Session

You may feel pretty good after a massage, but you also may feel sore later.

It's important to drink water after a massage. Why? To help hydrate the now flexible muscle fibers and to assist the removal of waste from the system.

Massage may make you have to use the bathroom.

If you're more sore than you want to be, it could help to ice the area. Massage therapy can make physical changes to your muscles and connective tissue. With change to the body comes soreness, from positive and negative changes both.

If you were too sore after your last massage, give that feedback to your therapist. If your therapist understands the outcome of your last massage, they can adjust the session to make it better for you.

Most massage therapists will probably try to get you to stretch on your own time.

After a good massage, stretching your muscles should be a little easier with less resistance and it's encouraged to gain more flexibility with the now relaxed muscles.

If you do *not* stretch after a massage, your muscles could creep back into those tight positions quicker than you want them to. Stretch to improve your flexibility.

Tip #7: Don't treat massage therapy like a toughness challenge.

Receiving a massage should be helpful. If the technique or pressure is too much, the muscles cannot relax. Your muscles will actually tighten if the massage pressure is too heavy or painful. Speak up when things are uncomfortable.

If your muscles are actively tightening from discomfort during a massage, it may create more soreness and may not be very helpful. If you need lighter pressure, tell us.

We (therapists) want your session to have the best results.

THREE
Muscles

This section will help you to see your muscles with more understanding.

Muscles should be viewed and treated as teammates, with you being a knowledgeable and caring coach. A good coach recognizes where their team is weak and tunes the team members up to work better and function stronger together.

This is the same way we should approach our human bodies.

Massage therapy can help discover and assist tight, tender, and painful parts so we can better coach our muscle teams with as much information as possible.

Therapists help to make irritated or struggling muscles known to you, the body owner, so you can give these muscles the attention they need. More massage, stretching, strengthening, or just a more general workout routine.

Muscles *require* motion to stay able. As your muscles contract and relax they provide a pumping of blood action that shares oxygen, nutrients, and hydration with the muscle cells.

When you hold positions, blood is blocked out of tightened muscles making it difficult for blood flow to reach those constricted areas very well. When it comes time to release those long-held positions, the muscles sometimes do not relax well enough to allow blood to flow back in. It's also possible for inflammation to block out proper blood flow.

As we use our muscles, sometimes we gain inflamemation. Even our diet can affect how much inflammation we build or hold onto.

Eating proper foods can remove excess inflammation from the body, making it easier for our functions.

We need to eat well and keep our muscles strong for them to have the best future possible. There aren't any good qualities to weak muscles.

3.1: MUSCLE HELP

Objects that help the muscles recover from tension or pain are used by millions of people in discomfort and pain every day. Solving a little discomfort today can protect your tomorrow from a deeper pain.

These helpful devices can assist with small daily discomforts. The results vary for each person. Use every piece of equipment how it was designed for maximum benefit and safety.

Ball Therapy

Use of a sports ball to apply pressure to tight or tender muscles.

- Tennis ball, baseball, lacrosse ball, golf ball: good for neck, back, and shoulder muscles. Try them on the feet also.
- Basketball: good to roll on the back and leg muscles to apply pressure for some relief.

Neck Pillows

This small pillow surrounds the neck, allowing for better neck resting support. People use these the most during travel.

Braces

Arm, leg, and back braces are commonly used for support and help the muscles to feel less struggle, which allows for them to be used easier. Neck braces are used for specific neck injuries, which falls under the "don't move it" rule of injured body parts.

Foam Rollers

Tough, compressed foam material, usually in a cylinder shape. Some come with knobs or "spikes" that give a harder pressure. The roller can help to relax tightened muscles and may assist with inflammation removal.

Similar to ball therapy, foam rollers can give more broad pressure to back and leg muscles.

Be careful not to put pressure on the spine or other bones. The foam roller is designed for muscular use.

Frozen Water Bottle

Good to roll your feet on if they have inflammation or pain. The rolling motion helps to stretch the foot material and the ice helps the inflammation to recede.

Ointments, Creams, Salves

For painful areas, it can be helpful to try a cooling type of cream or lotion.

Biofreeze is a good obvious example, but there are other brands or types that could help as a cold replacement. These ointments are quick to apply and helpful if you don't have time to use an ice pack.

There are so many pain cream options out there for sore muscles. Some may work better than others.

Always wash your hands after handling a muscle cream, ointment, or salve.

Tip #8: Some help is better than no help.

TENS Unit

Aka Transcutaneous Electrical Nerve Stimulation.

Sticky pads are placed on the desired muscle groups. The device sends small electrical currents into the pads causing the muscles to contract and relax rapidly. Always use caution and follow the instructions with any device.

Tip #9: If it hurts, stop doing it. (A classic tip)

Ask your doctor if you have concerns or questions about using health devices. It always helps to know more.

3.2: THE WORLD OF TENSION

This section will explain muscular tension. If you know what levels of tension you are working with, it's easier to manage them.

Tension forms in muscles and around joints that are <u>overused</u>, <u>underused</u>, <u>stressed</u>, <u>injured,</u> and <u>posture</u> holders. As you feel pain or stress, the muscular tension can increase. This will affect more muscle groups causing them to restrict mobility, strength, and stability as time goes.

To be more specific, muscle tension is when a group of muscle fibers hold their muscular contraction and are unable to release fully on its own.

It can be possible for low levels of tension to go away with some rest, exercise, and stretching. Once your muscles reach a high level of tension, stretching and other normal methods of muscular relief are far less helpful than they used to be.

Massage therapy can assist the muscles in releasing their tense state so that you can stretch and keep your muscular mobility strong through life.

Tension and stress are big reasons for raised blood pressure. With greater amounts of each, it's more likely that the heart can be affected.

Think of trying to drink a thick milkshake with a thin straw, it's very frustrating trying your hardest to get just a little milkshake through the straw. Why is it so hard to enjoy a milkshake!? *ahem*

That frustration is also what the heart feels when trying to squeeze blood through thin spaced arteries and extra tightened muscular groups.

According to the Centers for Disease Control, having uncontrolled hypertension (high blood pressure) puts you at risk for heart disease and stroke, which are leading causes of death in the United States.

Not the best news, but it's still important to know.

3.3: TENSION CHART

This is a visual guide to see where you stand on the tension chart. This will share the idea that certain levels of tension and stress can cause damage the longer you experience them. You want to be around the green area. Green is good.

Massage therapy can help you to climb the chart back towards green, as well as consistent self-care.

Ranging from no pain, no tension: Green healthy color (top, Level 1).

To heavy pain, severe muscle or joint damage: Dark red (bottom, Level 6).

The red is the danger zone. Time spent in the red zone can cause permanent joint damage.

TENSION CHART

Level 1 - Normal muscle ability and function.
No pain.

Level 2 - Some tension, some discomfort.
Light headaches.

Level 3 - Tension, discomfort.
Tight muscles lead to stiffness,
some headaches.
Sleep issues begin.

Level 4 - Tension with some pain, sticky connective tissue.
Headaches more often, stiff muscles.
Uncomfortable holding positions for long.
Losing some ROM.
Can't sleep well, mood can be affected.

Level 5 - Constant pain, serious tension,
frequent headaches, stiff muscles progressed to stuck muscles.
Motion resistant connective tissue, loss of ROM,
Can't sleep well, affected mood/temper.
Uncomfortable very often, hard to find relief.
Could cause emotional distress from losing physical ability.
Joint damage, excess inflammation build.

Level 6 - Same as the red zone but in the long term, could lead to permanent joint or
spine damage, leading to surgery.

Level 1: No tension/stress. – green

Level 2: Some tension, some discomfort. Light headaches. - yellow/green

Level 3: Tension, discomfort, tight muscles may lead to stiffness, some headaches. Sleep issues begin. -

Level 4: Tension with some pain, stuck connective tissue, headaches more often, stiff muscles, uncomfortable holding positions for long, losing some ROM, can't sleep well, and mood can be affected. - orange

Level 5: Constant pain, serious tension, frequent headaches, stiff muscles progressing to stuck muscles, less flexible connective tissue, loss of ROM, can't sleep well, affected mood/temper, uncomfortable very often. Could cause emotional distress from losing physical ability, joint damage, and excess inflammation build. - red

Level 6: Same as above, but in the long term. Could lead to permanent joint or spine damage, leading to surgery. - dark red

---

This is a visual representation of how I view the dangers of tense muscles. If you know where you stand on the chart, it can help you see that you may need to make some physical changes to improve and move towards the green zone.

Massage therapy is best utilized in the green zone to keep happy, healthy bodies on a happy and healthy path.

Massage can assist every zone on the chart, even after surgeries (Level 6).

It takes longer to correct the body in the higher levels of tension, but changes can still be made with good effort and a supportive care team.

Tip #10: Stay out of the red zone.   ← Goes along with the tension chart.

3.4: WHY DO WE GET TENSE?

Here are some reasons that our muscles get tense. More tension stuff, yay.

All of this is to help you know your body so that you can understand how to assist it the best. If you see yourself in these descriptions, it's time to make a good positive change. With a little effort and understanding, we can lessen the effects of tension.

Overuse

Overuse of muscles can cause tension, stiffness, soreness, pain, and inflammation. Prolonged overuse can lead to injury, dysfunction, weakness, loss of stamina, and damage to the joints.

Joint damage could lead to surgery.

Another way to describe **overuse** is: using the muscles beyond what their strength, flexibility, and stamina allows for consistent use. Overuse can create muscle micro-tearing which can cause consistent inflammation and scar tissue build, leading to stuck fascia (adhesions.)

Just remember, using both sides of your body equally could help to reduce some overuse or strain. Try to activate the non-dominant side a little more to create better muscular balance between both sides.

Repetitive strain problems are born from overuse. Mostly, it's caused by unevenly used, overused, or poorly rested muscle tissue.

It's difficult to rest hurting body parts and it takes time to recover. Put effort and understanding towards your body's situation.

Long term overuse can create dense layers of scar tissue and adhesions, which leads to restriction of motion and possible pain. More about scar tissue later.

Underuse

Underuse can cause poor muscular stability for the skeleton and extra wear on joints that are not properly supported. The stronger muscle groups have to work harder to allow the weaker muscles some stability or motion.

Muscular imbalance can make the entire skeleton's job more difficult.

Massage therapy can assist underused body parts by providing extra circulation, which is needed.

Example: Bed-ridden people are good candidates to receive massage to assist blood flow to unused muscles.

Stress

Stress is when the physical, mental, or emotional self meets with resistance. When stress builds and remains unaddressed, it can cause muscular tension, headaches, back pain, difficulty sleeping, and general discomfort. It can also affect the clarity of mind, mood, and temper.

Over time, stress can hurt the heart.

Massage is well known for helping to reduce stress and its effects on the human body and mind. Relaxing massage is most helpful if performed regularly to keep the effects of stress low.

With long term tension from stress, perhaps a deeper massage may be more helpful.

Injuries

Any force that causes the body to go through a deep healing process. Injuries can range from skin and muscle damage to broken bones and amputations.

Injuries can take from a couple weeks up to six months to heal *with proper treatment.* Yikes, I know.

Many injuries are earned through our jobs, hobbies, and accidents. Car accidents can cause a wide variety of injuries to the muscles and skeleton. Best to be avoided. Drive safely, please.

It takes a while for the human body to heal from each scenario we put it through. With knowledge, we can protect our bodies better.

Ask your doctor if you can get your injury massaged, they can help you make that decision.

Massage therapy can be helpful after any swelling has lessened.

Old injuries can usually be addressed with massage, too.

3.5: ADVANCED MUSCULAR TENSION

I believe there is a level of tension beyond normal everyday tension that I call Advanced Muscular Tension, or "Stuck muscles."

This is a higher level of muscular tension that has spread to a few layers of muscles and limits the affected region of the body's full ROM (Range of Motion) or strength.

Even the skin can be stuck down to these areas keeping the area dehydrated and restricted of blood and mobility.

I consider advanced muscular tension to be tension x2 or x3.

There are several reasons why your muscles resist motion or get stuck in place:

- Dehydration
- Long term overuse
- Long term underuse
- Long term position holding
- Untreated injury
- Long term guarding
- Surgery

Massage therapy can help reduce the effect that extra tense muscles have on the body, but it may take several sessions to make a big difference or a long-lasting change, especially with long term issues.

Just try to think of how much time has been spent gaining the issue. It will take some time to make a physical change, but progress can still be made.

3.6: INFLAMMATION

A word so many people hear and use. It's hard to imagine what exactly it is just from hearing it. The immune system is responsible for the production of this necessary healing material.

Inflammation is mostly made up of white blood cells and plasma from the blood. Its job is to put up a construction barricade and seal the damaged area off to allow healing to take place. The white blood cells use the plasma as its set up area to begin healing the damaged tissue.

Think of a police barricade set up to keep civilians out while an investigation happens. This is similar to how inflammation from damage works.

Prolonged Inflammation could cause excessive scar tissue build-up and sensitivity to touch, pressure, or motion.

Important: Inflammation has the ability to grow more than it should. This can cause even more soreness and pain. You can usually reduce some swelling by applying ice to the area or following the R.I.C.E (Rest, Ice, Compression, Elevation) guidelines. More about R.I.C.E in the Injury Zone.

Each and every time you work your muscles to the point of soreness or pain, your muscles create inflamemation to heal irritated and partially torn muscle fibers. If the overused area is not addressed with some form of relief or therapy, the repeated growth and cooling of the inflammation could bind the affected muscles with scar tissue, a little bit each time the event happens.

By not treating the small injuries as we get them, we are slowly creating stuck muscle and scar material. It's difficult to notice how these small problems affect us until we've created so many small stuck muscle groups, that our muscle function is noticeably or painfully restricted.

Tip #11: Reduce swelling and inflammation growth early.

3.7: How Massage Relates to Inflammation

Always be careful of inflamed body parts. Healing is occurring. Only light massage is recommended.

If the area is *highly* inflamed, It is not recommended for massage therapy. The surrounding areas can still be relaxed to assist drainage of excess inflammation.

Take care not to upset the inflammation growth with deep massage or repeated use of the affected region. Rest as much as the injury requires.

Avoid massage in bruises and swelling. Massaging bruises or swelling may increase inflammation and could damage the active healing process.

Your bruises need to heal some and your swelling needs to go down before massage can be helpful in those areas.

Ice is helpful to lessen inflammation. Your massage therapist can help work the affected area as soon as the inflammation levels come down.

Light massage therapy can help to flush out inflammation. As your circulation increases from receiving light massage, your body is able to eliminate the extra fluid more efficiently.

Massage with light pressure could make you have to use the bathroom. This is a good thing. That means things are moving.

3.8: SCAR TISSUE

The human body creates scar tissue to replace damaged material. Massage and physical therapy can aid the formation of scar tissue.

Inflammation begins the healing process and scar tissue forms to complete the healing process.

Massage can help improve a scar's formation as it heals and can assist the scar tissue to become more flexible. Some scar tissue can overgrow causing issues internally and/or externally and could also bind the connective tissues or muscles down. That's not good and not how you want your injuries to turn out.

After a surgery heals, massage can help the scar from the incision to recover better.

Burn scars can be assisted after the skin is healed. With burn scars, the region could be extra sensitive or numb to pressures and temperatures. Communicate with the therapist about anything uncomfortable that you feel.

The goal of scar massage is to keep the scar tissue from doing whatever it pleases and guide it to proper alignment and function.

Tip #12: Be thoughtful of all injuries.

3.9: INJURY ZONE

This section explains injuries and how they may be assisted with massage therapy. Everyone has the possibility of becoming injured. What's important is making sure the injured parts recover well.

Types of injuries:

Sprain

Overstretching or tearing of a ligament. Light massage can be helpful with **caution**. You don't want to make more inflammation trying to help the issue. Self-massage to the sprain is easier because you just want to give it a little attention without irritating it. An entire massage session may be too much for a new sprain.

Strain

Damage to the muscle or tendon. Often referred to as a pulled muscle. When swelling recedes, massage can be very helpful.

Hyperextension

Extending a joint past its available range of motion (ROM). Causes overstretched tendons and uncomfortable pressure in and around the joint. Massage can relax the area after any swelling fades.

Broken Bones

Recovery time can range from four to six weeks. Some bone breaks take longer. When your doctor says it is ok to get a massage, the sooner the better.

Massage can assist the muscles around the affected bone to relieve much stiffness of the muscle fibers that couldn't move during the healing process. It can also assist the muscles that performed extra support during the broken bone issue.

Burns

When burns heal, massage can help the scar tissue to improve. The therapist should use caution working over newly formed skin. A burn can affect the nerves, causing sensitivity or lack of feeling. Caution is recommended.

ASSISTING INJURIES

It's easy to cause an injury to persist longer than it should. Injuries require rest and time, and possibly even physical therapy to recover correctly. The R.I.C.E (Rest, Ice, Compression, Elevation) method is used often with minor injuries.

Here is why these things are helpful.

Rest

Rest allows the body to be in a comfortable position,

activating as few muscles as possible. Resting the affected area helps to reduce the amount of pain felt and inflamemation produced from irritation.

The non-use of a painful area allows the healing cells to work smoother and faster. With fewer hurdles to overcome, healing can progress quickly.

Imagine trying to do your job and someone is blocking your way or putting more people in your small workspace that take your equipment. It's not very helpful for your work goal and it would make your job harder and take longer. In this case, your healing would go slower and take longer to repair the area.

Think of rest as giving your team time to recover for the next game in the series. The body needs rest like it needs food, air, and water. Massage therapy can assist the body to rest easier, allowing for deeper sleep and better recovery times.

Many patients have told me that they slept so much better after getting a massage. It's a wonderful feeling to sleep well and I want that for everyone.

<u>Example</u>: Laying your body down flat allows your postural muscles in your back and hips to rest. Sitting up to watch tv may not be as restful as we all want it to be since it requires some postural muscles to be active.

Tip #13: Do not continuously move your hurt parts.

Resting can become a difficult chore the longer you have to do it.

Ice

Icing an injury can help to keep inflammation from growing wildly. Less inflammation means less swelling. Ice may shorten the time required for the affected area to heal. It also reduces the feeling of pain and numbs the affected area. ← Positive things.

Try not to move the cold muscles after ice is applied. Let the cold do its job by not moving the affected region. Feeling less pain allows for better rest. Ice pairs well with rest.

What and how you feel matters. If you feel pain, your body responds to it with more tension.

Compression

Compression helps to keep inflammation from swelling the affected area beyond comfort. Use of a tight band or brace can be helpful during the swelling stage.

Example: Using a bandage wrap around a swollen knee. It restricts the knees motion and reduces inflammation's ability to grow to uncomfortable levels.

Options for compression:

Pillow

If something is *very* tender even a little bit of pressure can be helpful within tolerance.

Weighted Blanket

Can range from 5 - 50 lbs. Helpful for keeping your sore areas from moving in an unwanted way while you sleep. Some people find the extra weight comforting.

Brace

Provides minor protection to the affected area. Assists with motion restriction to keep the area from being used to irritation. Can be helpful during or after work or hobby. Braces are made for feet, ankles, legs, back, arms, wrists, and neck.

Bandages

Can be wrapped around almost any part of the body manually. Mummies approve of these.

Be cautious when wrapping bandages, always start from the furthest end of the limb and wrap towards the heart. If too tight, release some of the bandage. You still need blood to get through there.

Elevation

Elevation pertains mostly to arms and legs. It isn't very easy to elevate the ol' torso. Resting the limbs in an elevated position allows the excess inflammation to drain away easier. Also, it helps to reduce the amount of swelling that settles in the affected area.

Additional Thoughts

Some injuries can require physical therapy, or even surgery to heal correctly. Proper treatment of a surgery is <u>extremely</u> important.

Untreated injuries could create permanent damage or dysfunction due to improper healing and scar tissue binding.

Tip #14: Patience should be practiced with all injuries.

Healing from an injury is a challenge.

Remember: You will always have things to do in life, but you only have a small window of opportunity to hurt or help your healing process. Choose to help your body in all cases. It's *your* body. Essentially, your brain's vehicle. Let your brain be proud of its ride.

When you damage your own healing process, it can cause dysfunctional healing. The scar tissue or adhesions can bind down on the muscles, connective tissue, or nerves in uncomfortable or painful ways over time. Most of us don't know this happens until it affects how we feel or move.

Massage therapy can help injuries as they heal and after they've healed.

Important: Check with your doctor to assess the state of an injury before getting any damaged area massaged.

Tip #15: The moment you lose mobility or function is when your life begins to change negatively, if you let it.

In most cases, we have a choice in how much time and effort we put into our own recovery. I believe, If you know more, you can do more to heal.

That's my whole purpose for this book. I don't want anyone to suffer if there is an obtainable solution.

With my life being affected by long-term damage, I strive to help others avoid the same issues. In my opinion, we can all treat ourselves and each other a little better.

3.10: PAIN

Everyone knows pain on some level. Physical, mental, or emotional. The response our body makes to pain varies by person. Some of us are crippled by it and others barely notice it. This is the pain perspective.

Pain is the alarm signal that lets the human body know something negative is happening to it and it's up to us, the body owner, to reduce the cause of the pain.

<u>Short story</u>:

Setting: Control room of a ship.

"Something is happening to the left foot, Captain Brain!" Left Leg Nerve announced.

"Aye, Lefty," Captain Brain said. "It is."

"Are you going to do something about it, sir?" Left Leg Nerve asked.

Captain Brain turned around, facing away from his crew. "I'll think about it," he said and allowed the body to limp forward.

Meanwhile the Left Leg Nerve struggled with the operation of the Left Leg Station.

When a human feels pain, muscular tension is created, even in areas where the pain is not directly located. The body responds to pain by automatically tightening the muscles for protection or *guarding*.

Guarding is what your muscles do when you feel pain or if your body perceives incoming pain, like a punch or object being thrown at you. Your muscles tense for protection.

Examples:

- With a headache, your neck and shoulder muscles could get tighter.
- If someone you care about goes through hardship, it can also affect your muscles through stress.
- If you stub your toe on a table or doorway. Many muscle groups all the way up to your neck could tighten up with tension. You also might hold your breath, which tightens muscles as well.

Most people can't feel that their muscles have tightened up until the affected muscles get to a level of tension that limits function, ability, or comfort.

Adding massage therapy to your life helps to lower your pain levels by relaxing the muscles and convincing your body to produce endorphins, the feel-good hormone. These hormones help to fight against cortisol, the hormone related to pain and our body's fight or flight response.

Tip #16: Address the pains as they appear and they could be easier to deal with.

It's *much* easier to recover from some physical tension rather than full blown injuries.

Injuries require time, rest, rehabilitation, and money for months possibly, whereas muscular tension requires much less effort, money, time, worry, and pain to overcome.

If you're experiencing pain and can't understand it well, a good massage therapist can help to assess the area and explain whether it's swollen, tight, hot to the touch, or restricted. If the problem is something outside of massage therapy's ability to help, we will refer you to your physician or another therapy.

If you have a concern for an ongoing pain, it's good to start with your family doctor to find out what your next step should be.

In many health journeys, it helps to have the right mindset to heal correctly. I believe you should listen to your body. No pain should be ignored for, eventually, it will grow and become louder until it has <u>all</u> of your attention.

Short story:

A young child asks his mom a question repeatedly while she's on an important phone call. The child is slowly getting louder with each repeat of the question.

The mother can't tune the child out anymore

and she can't hear the person on the phone either.

She's irritated because she can't focus on the call, but she doesn't want to be angry with the child because he's just being a normal quizzical kid.

"Are you mad at me?" the child asks.

"I'm not mad at you. I just can't hear Aunt Judy on the phone," the frustrated mom replies.

The point of this silly story is:

Tip #17: Your pains can keep you from focusing on your goals and only paying attention to them.

Please, don't let that happen.

3.11: HIGH PAIN TOLERANCE

High pain tolerance is the ability to feel pain and mentally push it away or to not feel pain correctly due to a nerve or other issue. This section will help you to understand what to be wary of if you or someone you know falls into this category.

Many people have the ability to shrug off heavy pains. I've met some incredible people with high pain tolerance. Some of us earn pain tolerance through receiving pain over a long period of time and some are born with it.

As a high pain tolerance person, your nerves tell you pain is happening, but you make a choice not to listen to it unless, of course, your nerves have a dysfunction, and you actually don't feel it.

A tolerance for deep or continuous pain can be dangerous to a person's body. The human body has a physical limit whether you can handle the pain feelings or not. Our mind may overcome the painful feelings, but the body still has to deal with the effects.

Damage is still being done and it still needs to be treated. Damage is damage, inflammation is still being sent to help the damaged area. You may be able to mentally curb how you react to the pain, but your body could be struggling harder than you realize. The body's functions and ability could be damaged eventually, which is something that can be avoided with understanding and proper care for the body.

High pain isn't very apparent to people that can handle the pain received. Most humans react to severe pain because it hurts and it's necessary for the system to feel less pain to be able to be used to its highest ability.

Pain is an alarm signal, exactly like a fire alarm. It's not a positive thing to experience for the long term. High Pain Tolerance (HPT) can be a negative thing if the body owner ignores those important alarms for extended amounts of time.

Imagine ignoring fire alarms. I don't like that scenario.

Also, imagine hearing fire alarms constantly. That's bad, too.

Tip #18: It becomes much easier to injure the body when pain is ignored or untreated.

With massage many people request deep pressure, which is perfectly fine and acceptable. It's important for the therapist to know where to draw the line when the request for pressure goes against their knowledge of the body.

Some regions of the body cannot handle as much pressure as some people may want.

<u>Example</u>: less pressure over the kidneys, ribs, lymph nodes, or known artery pathways.

Deep tissue massage doesn't mean it has to be the deepest pressure imaginable. You can have great deep tissue work with excellent results without using very deep pressures at all. When applied often and correctly, the deep tissue massage techniques help to make the greater difference.

When you have HPT, massage quality or results may be different for you. Just try to understand that through massage therapy, the muscular tissue is still being affected in a positive way even if you don't get pain feelings.

Some people have the belief of "no pain, no gain". I believe that to be true within reason. Be careful of all pain. Be aware of it and treat it well.

Tip #19a: Do not ignore your pain.

Tip #19b: Just because you *can* handle pain, doesn't mean you should.

If you feel something, do something. The same as if you laid your hand on a hot stove. MOVE IT! Don't just try to overcome the 4th degree burns with your mental will.

The damage that comes with ignoring pain is hard to measure and treat over the long term.

It might sound like a lot of negatives there, but I believe it's more about understanding any issue to a higher degree.

Massage therapy can be helpful on High Pain Tolerance clients with understanding on both sides, client and therapist.

Get massage therapy often to aid these small problems as they show up. Just remember, you don't have to be amazingly sore the next day for the massage to be helpful.

<u>FOUR</u>
Body Awareness and Posture

This section explains the idea of considering every body part as if it were important.

Body Awareness is understanding and using your body to a more knowledgeable degree. When we are aware of the state of our body's abilities and functions, we know what muscles or joints are tight, painful, weak, flexible, strong, or perfectly fine.

Being body aware allows us to comprehend any negative changes to the body. This allows us to deal with the physical issue before it settles in as a deeper problem.

Having good body awareness is like taking your car into the shop when you notice an issue at the first sign, instead of waiting for several problems to build up first.

Tip #20: Do something positive for the small issues you feel on a daily basis.

Body Awareness can be practiced by feeling each part

of your body and moving each joint, one at a time. Similar to washing with a cloth in the shower, touch each part of your body with your hands or your thoughts. Take time to understand what each portion of your body is feeling and going through.

<u>Example</u>: Think of your feet and focus on them. Are they in pain? Do they move? Can they perform every motion you need them to? Are they restricted at all?

You move every moveable component and assess it, then you continue with your ankles, moving one at a time and so on until you complete your analysis of your body.

It takes some time to do a full assessment of yourself. Break it up into several different sessions. Create a routine with it. This method can show you if any body parts are having problems.

Being body aware can give you a heads up to get massage therapy or some other type of care before the problem gets worse.

When you are aware of your body, it's much easier to determine the type of massage session that you need. A good massage therapist can help your body awareness improve with therapeutic touch.

Awareness!

Tip #21: Be aware and give care.

4.1: THE WHYS OF POSTURE

This section clarifies the needs for good posture and why it's important to start at a young age.

Holding correct postures starting in our youth helps to build necessary supportive postural muscles along the spine and in the core.

Building your back strength little by little as we get heavier over our growth periods is much easier than needing to build a lot of strength in weak muscles later on as an adult.

When a parent repeatedly tells their child to sit up straight, it helps it to become a habit. Many humans don't use proper posture because their muscles aren't able to be used consistently.

Tip #22: Using weak muscles can bring some pain.

When weak muscles are challenged by necessity, they are forced to act at their mightiest and that can bring pain, soreness, and inflammation.

Where weak muscles have to use almost 100% of their strength to accomplish their task, strong muscles can work easier with less pain.

Building core muscles in and around the abdomen assists the low back with its supportive job. The more you think about holding the correct posture, the more you do it. Try to keep posture in mind.

As an adult, if you haven't held good posture, it's

possible that some muscular weakness or imbalance isn't supporting your spine correctly.

Getting uncomfortable while you're sitting could mean your muscles are tired of holding position, holding improper posture, or responding to an unsupportive chair. Another possibility is spinal misalignment, but that's for a chiropractic doctor to determine.

Do you change positions often as you sit for periods of time? Leaning left, leaning right, shifting your hips, crossing legs, or pulling your legs up underneath you as you sit.

Massage can relax the postural muscles so they can support with less resistance. When tension holds in our posture, it reduces the muscles' stamina.

Tip #23: Strong, flexible muscles can endure more and perform better than overly tight, overused muscles.

Holding postures can continuously aggravate a back issue, leading to inflammation and decreased stability. Over time, postural muscles can lose their ability to support, becoming rigid and less responsive.

<u>Example</u>: Assembly line workers bending over for eight to ten hours out of the day to complete a portion of their job.

Massage therapy can relax postural muscles, allowing them to release from the repetitively held position. This will help the muscles to perform their job better, for longer, and with less complaint.

Muscles need regular motion to provide the best

blood flow to keep all the cells fed with blood, oxygen, nutrients, and hydration.

Even excellent functioning posture with good blood flow cannot overcome poor equipment over the long term.

This leads us back to Tip #4: **Use the right tool for the job.**

4.2: EQUIPMENT

Being comfortable in work positions is not only smart, but important. When it's time to change or upgrade equipment, remember that it's worth it. Some equipment can wear down and needs to be replaced so our bodies don't pay the price.

Use ergonomics in every work setting to reduce the damage you receive from the job.

Ergonomics

Efficient equipment placement to reduce operator fatigue and injury. This is important for anyone that uses equipment at work. Being ergonomic can reduce wear and tear on the body, by using equipment that works for you.

Be aware of how equipment affects your body and make the changes necessary.

Chair

A work chair should be comfortable and easy to hold correct posture. Improper chair height can bring pressure to legs and could cause numbness or lack of blood flow to legs or feet.

<u>Example</u>: sitting for six hours, you may notice you're chilly. The reason could be that you haven't moved for many hours. Moving blood creates warmth through the

system.

Desk Type

Desks must be a comfortable height so you can use posture correctly and comfortably. Goes well with a supportive chair. A stand-up desk offers your muscles a different position than only sitting.

Computer Monitor

Keep your monitor at eye level so you're not looking up or down. Your neck should be relaxed as you use the computer.

Headset

A headset is used for communications jobs, eases neck stress and tension. Your headset should be comfortable and light.

Phone

Phone overuse can cause uneven tension to the neck and possibly cause a strain to one side of the neck.

Over time, phone usage may affect the alignment of the spine in the neck, which could cause muscular tension and pain.

Tool Belt

Tool belts can become very heavy and will eventually affect the hips and back.

Backpack

Many jobs have equipment that people wear on their back. These packs can weigh on the back, creating pain and tension. Students, bug sprayers, landscapers, and flamethrowers.

Additional Thoughts

An injury from using equipment is called a Musculoskeletal Disorder (MSD).

The key to proper posture is the position of your spine. Your head should be above your shoulders, and your shoulders should be over the hips.

Lean forward or backward just a little too far and you are no longer in proper posture.

The muscles associated with any work equipment could improve with the benefits of massage therapy.

4.3: Long-Term Bad Posture

The issues with bad posture can remain hidden until the breaking point has been reached. The last straw that broke the camel's back is a common comparison with this. Our bodies are capable of incredible things, but there is always a limit to what it can endure.

Every muscle cell needs access to blood (Oxygen, hydration, nutrients, and vitamins), but tight or restricted muscles receive less blood.

When you hold poor posture for an extended amount of time, the muscles are being used in a way that they are not designed for. Over time, bad posture can cause supportive muscles to become weak and lose the ability to support properly.

The benefits of massage will help your muscles become more flexible and supportive again.

Tip #24: Each effort you put towards your health journey matters.

<u>Example</u>: Slouching. It's incredibly easy for people to slouch if their backs are weak, tired, overused, under-developed, or in pain. This position can restrict chest and shoulder muscles, holding them in a forward position.

The neck struggles when it's not sitting directly over the spine. Eventually, slouching can cause spinal issues from the neck to the low back.

The spinal bones protect the spinal cord where the

nerves extend from. Keep the spine happy, keep the nerves happy, keep the muscles happy. There's a pattern here.

<u>Examples of the effects of long-term bad posture</u>:

- Disrupts proper spinal alignment
- Headaches
- Difficulty holding proper posture
- Back problems
- **Early arthritis onset**

It's difficult to use good posture if your muscles aren't ready to support that positional hold consistently. A good thing to remember is that massage therapy can assist muscles during the strengthening phase too.

4.4: CORE IMPORTANCE

Core muscles complete the support that the back requires. An engaged core creates a circle of supportive strength. Strong core muscles help to reduce back strain.

The core consists of abdominal, side abdominals, and other midsection muscles that stabilize your spine, ribs, and pelvis.

<u>Fun Note</u>: Core muscles can be engaged at any time. **They can be activated as you sit at a desk or in a car. You can work your core as you walk too.**

The back muscles have a big job and the core stabilizes it as it works. A weak core isn't able to assist the back and causes muscular struggle the longer the back muscles work alone.

Imagine being a blue triceratops at the bottom of a dino-pyramid. You are placed in the bottom middle underneath everyone else. The people next to you aren't supporting the people above them. All the weight of the pyramid comes down on you and only you for support.

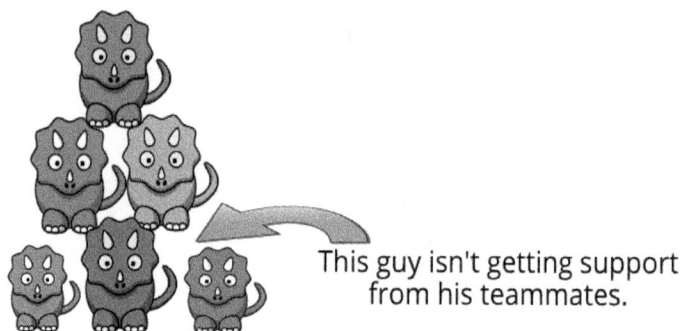

This guy isn't getting support from his teammates.

Now, the bottom of the pyramid is unhappy. That's not how we want our pyramids or our backs to be.

The core muscles are like the back's savior.

Tip #25: Be core strong to save your back from struggle.

If you really want to change a physical issue, you **must** give it attention and tend to what is causing the dysfunction.

Better posture is achievable, and you can make it happen.

4.5: Holding Positions

We all have to hold positions with our bodies for work, family, or hobby.

Holding positions for long periods can cause the muscles to become overused, tense, tired, stiff, and weak. Prolonged holding of positions for weeks, months, or years can negatively impact the human body.

Massage reduces the problems associated with holding positions and makes it easier to continue to perform those positions.

Position examples:

- Standing
- Sitting
- Looking down/up
- Bending over
- Squatting
- Twisting
- Overhead reaching

All of these positions can improve with massage therapy.

It's good to have a deeper understanding of the motions that you make at work or play. If you *know* what body parts are your work tools, the next step is to know how to assist those muscles to stay functional and healthy.

Massage therapy can assist muscles that you use every day. Giving overused muscles the opportunity for massage could allow for greater longevity with your motions.

It all boils down to, Massage therapy should be kept in your self-care routine to allow for long lasting physical ability.

Final word about positions: Be mindful of your positions and how long you hold them.

4.6: MUSCULAR STIFFNESS

Stiffness is a little different than tension. It's created from holding positions usually. You gain tension over the long run, but it can all start with a little stiffness and worsen from there.

We gain tension by overusing our muscles for action, feeling pain over time, and stress.

Stiffness most often comes from holding a position for such an amount of time that when you go to change your position the muscle doesn't want to let go. It could also come from repeated heavy lifting or continuous muscle use without engaging in a proper cooldown.

Examples:

- Sleeping in an awkward position
- Aggressive workout
- Holding positions for too long
- Some muscles may get stiff as a side effect of medication.

No matter the cause, massage therapy can help reduce muscular stiffness.

Example: You're sitting down in a chair for thirty minutes. It's time to get up and do something. Standing up, your back has a hard time relieving the sitting posture. Usually, this motion is accompanied by an "Ohhhh" or some other general groan. We all groan differently.

This is a perfect example of stiff muscles.

The human body doesn't like to sit for a long time unless those muscles are healthy, strong, supportive, and able to move correctly. Even with strong healthy muscles, they still need to be relieved of their position regularly.

Holding muscles in a contracted state limits how much blood can get into the held muscles. Motion brings blood which brings nutrients, oxygen, and hydration.

You know what? I think I'm going to make that into a tip.

Tip #26: Muscles require motion to be healthy.

When stiff muscles are massaged, the recipient can feel a tender or sensitive feeling at first. After a couple minutes of warming up the affected area with massage techniques, the tenderness usually reduces and deeper pressure could be applied if desired.

Regular exercise provides increased blood flow, which feeds and fuels all of the cells that the blood comes in contact with.

Tip #27: No blood, no life. ← It sounds harsh but it's true.

This tip refers to restricted muscles that are unable to receive blood well.

Imagine this:

- A whale on a shore needs water. ←-You just know it does.

114

- A person underwater needs air. ←-You absolutely know that a person needs to breathe air.
- A muscle kept from motion is like a whale on a shore or a person underwater. It needs what it breathes, which is blood. Without blood flow comes restriction or ischemia (lack of blood flow).

Blood = Oxygen, hydration, and nutrition.

No motion = No blood = No food for the cells = Poor cell health.

Muscle cells specifically require calcium, potassium, vitamin D, and magnesium to contract and relax properly.

Massage therapy can move blood into stiffened muscle material to help it to relax, flush out overstayed inflammation, and break up scar tissue. Blood can enter into the relaxed muscles, which allows better nutrient absorption and waste removal.

Your muscles use blood to flex, extend, move, breath, heal, and to be alive. Think of the difference between bending a dry sponge and wet sponge. The wet sponge bends and the dry sponge breaks.

4.7: RELAXATION

The body and mind make up an incredible team that allows amazing ability if you maintain your physical and mental health. Relaxation is a key component to keep our human bodies able and well. Here are some easy ways to relax.

Massage Therapy

During a massage session, relaxing music helps with letting stress go. A comfortable massage setting with a trusted therapist can help the body and mind relax on a deep level.

As massage therapy techniques are applied, the human body can produce the "feel good" hormone, endorphins, which aids relaxation.

<u>Fun Note</u>: Laughing can also create a surge of endorphins.

Breathing

Breathe deeper and more completely instead of taking short, shallow breaths. Inflating your lungs deeper during regular breathing allows for clearer thought and it actually assists with relaxing your muscles.

The human body requires oxygen, and we get it from breathing. Deeper breathing means more oxygen.

There are many moments in a person's day where we

may become focused and stop breathing smoothly.

Example: Focused on work, reading, driving, playing video games, watching movies, etc.

You may be holding your breath or be taking many short, shallow breaths. Holding our breath can cause muscular tension or stress to affect us deeper.

Remember to breathe more completely, even when you're very focused. It's absolutely something you can learn to do. I know you can do it!

Back, rib, chest, and neck muscles can restrict the ability to breathe deeply when they are affected with tension or stress.

Massage therapy can assist the muscles to allow deeper breathing.

Fun note: When a person sees the word breathe, they tend to take a deep breath. I bet you breathed deeper during this section than any of the others you've read.

Pleasant Smells

Pleasant smells are much more beneficial than bad smells. A bad smell can sour your mood, but pleasant smells can improve moods and make it easier to relax in your environment. Smelling a pleasant scent may encourage deeper breathing.

Examples:

- Candles
- Incense

- Clean living space
- Citrus

All pleasant smells. With a little thought, I'm sure you can find a smell that helps you to relax. Take the time to enjoy the smells that bring you closest to the state of relaxation.

Stretching

Stretching will help your muscles retain or regain their ability to relax and move with greater ease. Tense muscles won't change if they aren't encouraged.

Massage therapists are trained in some stretching. Ask questions and learn what stretches you can do to continue addressing your muscles daily.

You brush your teeth to prevent problems and to have good breath. Stretching does that, too, except for the good breath part.

After massage, stretching can be performed easier and will help to keep tension away.

Ahh, Relaxation. What is life without you?

4.8: BODY MATH

This device will help you see how well your body is doing on a daily, weekly, or monthly basis. The math that you do here will help you grasp your physical situation better.

After seeing how much and how often your negatives show up, that knowledge will allow you to make the changes that are needed to become increasingly positive through your days.

The selections below may only be counted once in a day. At the end of the day, write down each selection that affected you for the negative and positive sides.

Keep your positive and negative numbers separate. It's important to see both sides of the spectrum.

- - Negatives - -	Long term Negatives	+ + Positives + +
Things that make your body struggle.	*& Advanced Conditions*	*Things that help your body.*
-Overworked -15	-30	+Massage therapy +50
-Underworked -10	-18	+Being active, Gym +5/+10
-Not enough sleep -8	-16	+Sports +12

-Major Injury -50	-With broken bones -110	+Walk (15-30 mins) +6
-Minor Injury -15	-Many minor Injuries -40	+Vitamins +2
-Sick(e.g. Flu) -25	-50	+Stretch a little +4
-Headache -6	-Frequent headache -13	+Stretch more +10
-Migraine -15	-30	+Hydration +3
-Poor Posture -3	-6	+Good posture +2
-Stress -2	-6	+Deep breaths +2
-Poor diet -4	-8	+Good diet +3
-Pain -6	-12	+Epsom salt soak +10
-Too little walking -3	-Very little motion -10	
-Car accident -30	-Severe accident -65	
-Tension -5	-11	
-Surgery -30	-Multiple Surgeries -80	

There are more negative options and they hit harder than the positives. To make the biggest and best difference, the positives need to be completed consistently.

You can record your negatives and positives for a week, a month, or more. If you keep good records of your body math for an entire month you can begin to see how you are using your body and what you are actually doing to improve or hurt it.

Having a visual numerical value can help people understand themselves better and make improvements where needed.

If you disagree with my number system, you can change the values to how you feel it affects you and your life. You can also add your own positive and negative selections to the list above. Just be reasonable with the number values that you assign to them.

It can help to write a list of positives and negatives and keep it nearby to have a constant reminder to increase your positive output. Sometimes all we really need is a friendly reminder to get that boost to do better.

At the end of the day or week, total up your negative and positive numbers. If you're in the negative, that's ok. This can give you motivation to add some of the positive choices to your next day.

We're all going to have negatives in our life, but what matters is how much positive we put in to create balance.

4.9: BODY MATH CALENDAR

Here is a calendar to record your daily body math. Write your negative and positive totals in the same block, negative on left and positive on right.

For example, these are the negatives for my day. I did not use long term negative numbers: Overworked -15, not enough sleep -8, and headache -6.

These make up my positives: Stretch a little +4, walking +6, and good diet +3.

Write the negative and positive totals in the box for the day.

Today I came out negative. I'll do better tomorrow.

-29 +13

Here is your free body math calendar. Use this to write your body math in.

If you wanted to write your body math on something different, that's ok. Don't even give these boxes another thought. It's ok; go ahead to the last chapter.

<u>FIVE</u>
Final Thoughts

Some final thoughts, in conclusion.

Write Away

Feel free to write in this book like it's your personal notebook. Circle, underline, highlight, and bookmark. Share your favorite tips with your friends and loved ones. This book can work as a reminder that we can all keep making progress for the better.

Check Motions and Muscles

A human being should check the quality of all of their motions and muscles regularly.

Can you touch toes, squat, raise your arms up high, lift your legs high(marching), jump?

These are all general motions. The very moment you

notice that one of your abilities has reduced in any way is the time to correct the issue. Your body will appreciate it if you keep its ability and functions strong.

Getting massage therapy regularly helps to keep you aware of any tender changes as they appear, giving you a heads up on what needs more care, when to get the care, and why to get the care.

The more you know about your physical problem, the easier it is to find a solution.

Start Slow

Many people may read this and say, "I can't remember the last time I jumped."

Always be careful when adding anything new to your daily routine. It's easy to overdo new motions, especially with unhealthy or weak muscle tissue.

When performing a new or infrequent motion, your muscles may not respond as quickly or with as much strength as you want them to.

Balance

Maintaining equal strength on both sides of the body will help to support your spine and physical ability properly.

Keep your actions and musculature as balanced as you can. Balanced musculature may protect your muscles and joints from being overused unevenly.

If you realize that you are very one-sided. Left or

right. Now may be the time to try for balanced muscle.

Understanding your body better could possibly reduce repetitive injuries as long as you listen to the pain your body tells you about. Remember, pain is an alert signal to get you to act against the problem.

Reduce Pain and Dysfunction

Fighting through pain should only last for a short term. Use all possible options to reduce pain and dysfunction. Don't ignore your body or its struggles.

Dysfunction doesn't usually go away on its own. It can only get worse without assistance or care.

Ticklish?

Massage has been known to reduce some ticklish areas' sensitivities.

Massage therapy can be a challenge for *very* ticklish people. There are some methods that therapists use to reduce the ticklish effect, but people are ticklish to varying degrees and the techniques may not work for everyone.

Ticklish people still need care.

Chiropractic Care and Massage

Massage therapy and chiropractic care are a duo similar to peanut butter and jelly. They work together extremely well. When massage therapy relaxes the muscles, the chiropractor can adjust those bony segments with greater ease resulting in longer lasting results.

Some muscles need to be able to relax better before an adjustment can really have a great effect, especially if you've had an injury.

A well-rounded care team can help you through many trials in life.

Many people enjoy chiropractic care by itself, but when paired with regular massage, your results could be greater.

AFTERWORD

I want to thank everyone that has allowed me to practice and learn with them over the years. 10+ years in and hopefully 10+ more to come. Learning and sharing knowledge with my patients has been a blessing for me. Massage has even helped me to understand some of my own physical limitations and overcome them. Take care of yourself and keep working towards a pain free future.

Levi Eckert
December 6, 2023

<u>APPENDIX A</u>
TREASURE TROVE OF TIPS

A quick reference guide to your tips found in the text.

Tip #1: Treat the feet well.

Tip #2: Making your injured body parts struggle may not be helpful.

Tip #3: The more you know, the less you guess.

Tip #4: Use the right tool for the job.

Tip #5: Consistency is the key to noticeable change.

Tip #6: The ability of each massage therapist varies.

Tip #7: Don't treat massage therapy like a toughness challenge.

Tip #8: Some help is better than no help.

Tip #9: If it hurts, stop doing it. (A classic tip)

Tip #10: Stay out of the red zone. ← Goes along with the tension chart.

Tip #11: Reduce swelling and inflammation growth early.

Tip #12: Be thoughtful of all injuries.

Tip #13: Do not continuously move your hurt parts.

Tip #14: Patience should be practiced with all injuries.

Tip #15: The moment you lose mobility or function is when your life begins to change negatively, if you let it.

Tip #16: Address the pains as they appear and they could be easier to deal with.

Tip #17: Your pains can keep you from focusing on your goals and only paying attention to them.

Tip #18: It becomes much easier to injure the body when pain is ignored or untreated.

Tip #19a: Do not ignore your pain.

Tip #19b: Just because you *can* handle pain doesn't mean you should.

Tip #20: Do something positive for the small issues you feel on a daily basis.

Tip #21: Be aware and give care.

Tip #22: Using weak muscles can bring some pain.

Tip #23: Strong, flexible muscles can endure more and perform better than overly tight, overused muscles.

Tip #24: Each effort you put towards your health journey matters.

Tip #25: Be core strong to save your back from struggle.

Tip #26: Muscles require motion to be healthy.

Tip #27: No blood, no life. ← It sounds harsh. But it's true.

Levi's Phrases

- "If you don't have motion, you don't have much."
- "Motion is everything."
- "Some of that tension can creep back in if you don't stretch after a massage."
- "Remember to drink some extra water, and if you feel sore later, use some ice."
- "This isn't about whether you can handle the pain or not; this is about you not feeling the pain at all."
- "Woo, I finished my book!"

APPENDIX B
FREQUENTLY ASKED QUESTIONS

1. Do I need massage therapy?

Most likely, yes. If you play any sport, use the computer, play video games, watch tv, do yard work, perform a hobby, drive for any length of time, have an injury, or if you work at a job. Also, if you don't use your body very much at all, you could benefit from massage.

Some of the muscle systems could start to bind up and resist motion. Short-term small discomforts are much easier to relax and change than long term issues, but massage can still help in both cases.

If you are unsure if you should get massage therapy for a specific issue, ask your doctor to clear up any concerns.

2. Is it ok to be nervous about massage?

That's fine and normal. Many people are nervous or don't know what to expect with a massage. Ask a massage therapist questions to help ease your mind.

You can relax deeper with a therapist you can feel comfortable with or trust.

Some massage therapists schedule consultations to meet and answer questions. You can then decide if you feel comfortable and want to proceed. A consultation may come with a minor fee, depending on the therapist.

I hope that the information in this book will help to remove some of the hesitancy involved with entering the world of massage.

3. Do I take any clothes off for a massage?

Yes, you can, but you don't have to. You can undress to the level of your comfort. Sports clothing or flexible fabric is best in my opinion.

Some people get fully nude to receive massage therapy and others may remain partially or fully clothed. Every patient or client is draped so no private area is exposed.

A massage works to its best without clothing hindering the massage techniques, but progress can still be made in any case.

Example: I'm shy. I take off as little clothing as I need to for a massage.

If you are comfortable, you will relax better. Even if that is lying fully clothed on a massage table.

If you are uncomfortable taking your clothes off, then try a chair massage session. The therapist most often focuses on the neck, shoulders, and upper back for one of these sessions. People usually remain fully clothed for a chair massage.

4. Can I have too much massage?

Yes. Eventually, the muscles, skin, and connective tissue becomes irritated, then damaged, and then bruised. Too much massage could result in inflammation, bruising, and pain.

5. Should I tip my massage therapist?

In most cases, yes. There are some businesses where tipping is discouraged or just not allowed. Just ask when you pay. Office staff can tell you if it's ok to tip.

I believe you should tip according to how much you appreciate your massage therapist and the work they did for you.

Was it wonderful? Did it meet your expectations or more? Did it make your day or week better? If so, share a tip up to 20% of your massage's cost.

Do you *have* to tip? No. You don't have to tip if you don't want to, although some spas or massage businesses may add a gratuity charge.

<u>GLOSSARY</u>

Adhesion

A band of scar tissue that can bind muscle ability or joint motion. This scar tissue can stick to other muscles or connective tissues that are not normally connected. Can hinder function.

Body Awareness

A continuous understanding of the state of your body.

Connective Tissue

Surrounds and supports bones, muscles, tendons, ligaments, and organs. This material holds everything together and in place. Some people use the term **fascia**.

Guarding

Muscles hold tension due to feelings of pain or threat of pain.

High Pain Tolerance (HPT)

The ability to push aside heavy pains with willpower or nerve dysfunction.

Injury

Any force that causes the body to go through a deep healing process.

Ischemia

Lack of blood flow to a part of the body.

Massage Therapy

Manipulation of soft tissues of the body (with hands or instrument) by a massage therapist. Therapeutic techniques are applied to the body to relieve pain, promote healing, and improve mobility.

Muscle

A soft tissue system made of cells that contract when stimulated. Produces motion.

Musculoskeletal Disorder (MSD)

Musculoskeletal disorders are injuries or pain in the bones, joints, ligaments, muscles, or tendons. These are often caused by repetitive strain or force injuries.

Range of Motion (ROM)
The limit to which a joint or appendage can move.

R.I.C.E.
Rest, ice, compression, elevation.

Self-Care
Anything that you do to improve your physical, mental, or emotional health.

Stress
When the physical, mental, or emotional self meets with resistance.

Trigger point (TP)
A tense knot of muscle that can affect the local nerves. May send a pain sensation with pressure.

ACKNOWLEDGMENTS

I would like to thank everyone who helped make this book become a reality. Your contributions may help people get the care that they need when they need it the most. Thank you eternally for being a part of this project:

Dawn Watson: Thank you for your support and every ounce of help from start to finish.

Dr. Brandy Chapman, Amy Hammond, Phyllis Bates: Thanks for looking over the material and helping to guide me along the way.

Juan Carlos Valverde: Thanks for helping me to broaden my thinking on my topics.

Greenville Tech's Massage Therapy Program: You changed my life more than I expected you would, and I'm happy for it.

Everyone at Carolina Spine and Health: Thanks for enduring my talk of making a book for so long.

Massage Therapists everywhere: Thank you all for choosing to care for people.

And all of the people that helped me to learn along the way.

Extra thanks to Sketch.IO. for sharing the triceratops.

And thank you, reader, for making it this far.

ABOUT THE AUTHOR

Levi G. Eckert grew up in the continuously growing city of Greenville, SC, and has practiced massage therapy since 2012. At the age of 23, he had an injury that sent him down the path of disability, pain, and physical recovery. He suffered from broken bones, head injury, and spinal nerve damage.

Eventually this path of pain brought him to college, a place he swore he would never go. He studied at Greenville Technical College in their massage therapy program (2011) where he made the Dean's list throughout the course.

Greenville Tech's Massage Therapy program was eye opening to Levi. He took it seriously due to his knowledge and experience in the world of physical pain and dysfunction.

Soon after becoming a licensed massage therapist, a classmate told him of a need for a therapist at a local chiropractor. He applied and was hired. Thus began his journey toward fighting against pain and dysfunction for others as well as himself.

He continues to enjoy his work of helping injured humans to recover and teaching them to understand their bodies better.

Contact Levi:
mythicpenprinting@gmail.com

Connect with Levi on Facebook to learn more about his work as a massage therapist and to discover the fictional worlds he creates for younger readers during his free time.

Facebook.com/LeviEckertAuthor

Join Flip, his best friend Trace, and their many friends on a magical journey as they protect their village from an unknown threat.

Flip's Quest
Coming soon

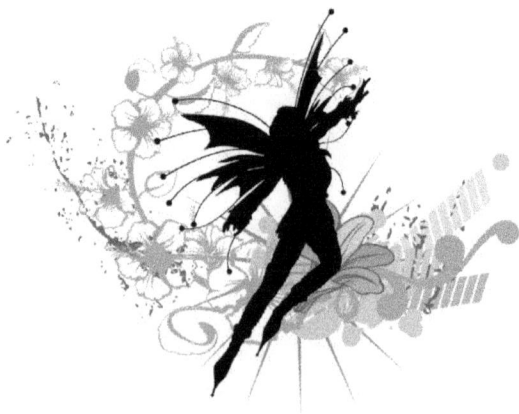

www.ingramcontent.com/pod-product-compliance
Lightning Source LLC
Chambersburg PA
CBHW060234030426
42335CB00014B/1458